Kegel Magic: A Comprehensive Guide to Effective Pelvic Floor Exercises for Men and Women

...maximizing sexual and urinary health...

Joel S. Lawson, M.D.

Table of Contents

INTRODUCTION

Kegel exercises is named after Dr. Arnold Kegel, who first developed these exercises in 1948. These exercises constitute the contraction and relaxation of the pelvic floor muscles. The pelvic floor muscles are essential for the support of several pelvic organs, the control of the bladder and intestine, and sexual function. Kegel exercises are designed to strengthen these muscles, which will improve general wellbeing, prevent or treat pelvic floor disorders, and promote better sexual experience.

This book, "Kegel Magic: A Comprehensive Guide to Effective Pelvic Floor Exercises for Men and Women" is your companion on the path to ideal pelvic floor health. The book uses a simple but thorough approach, and it promises to transform your pelvic floor muscles, thereby offering you a better control of your bladder and intestine, and a mind-blowing sex life. This book will advance your knowledge, proficiency, and use of Kegel exercises in your everyday life. It covers the following areas of interest:

- Foundations of understanding
- Personalized approach
- Step-by-step exercises
- Tailored guidance for women
- Tailored guidance for men
- Overcoming challenges
- Beyond Kegels: All-round wellness
- Monitoring progress and long-term success
- Integrating Kegels into daily life

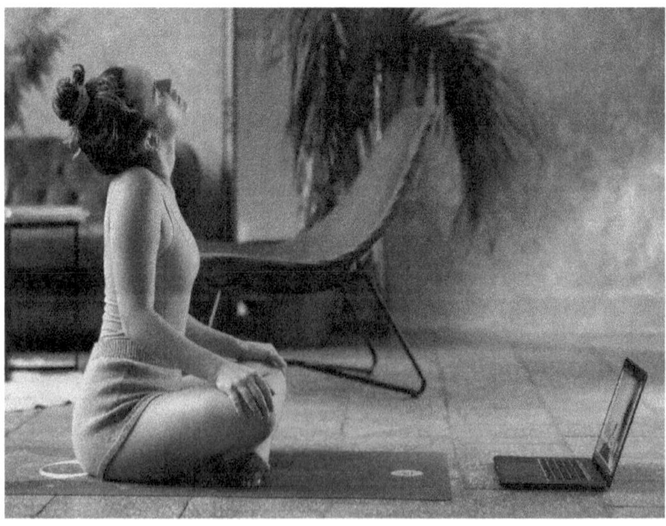

CHAPTER ONE

THE PELVIC FLOOR

A complex network of muscles, tendons, and ligaments makes up the pelvic floor and serves as the foundation for the pelvis, supporting numerous organs and facilitating many bodily functions. These muscles include the following:

Pubococcygeus Muscle (PC): It is situated near the base of the pelvis, encircling the anus, vagina, and base of the penis in a figure-eight pattern. It has a major role in controlling urine since it envelops the urethra. For both men and women, the PC muscle must be actively engaged in order to control the bladder and perform sexual functions.

Iliococcygeus Muscle: It extends from the ischial spine to the coccyx and aids in the pelvic organs' general support. It works along with the PC muscle to regulate fecal and urine continence. It takes active participation in maintaining the pelvic floor's stability during a range of motions.

Puborectalis Muscle: It helps to keep the rectum in a sling-like configuration, which aids in maintaining fecal continence. It is essential for preventing involuntary bowel leaking in the anorectal angle during bowel movements.

Perineal Muscles: It consists of a number of smaller muscles in the perineum, which is the region between the genitalia and the anus. They play an important function in preserving perineal integrity and supporting the pelvic organs. They contribute to sexual function and pleasure.

Functions of the pelvic floor

1. Pelvic Organ Support and Sustainment:

Vital pelvic organs like the bladder, uterus (in women), and rectum are held in place and supported by the pelvic floor, which functions as a hammock.

This structural support is essential in preventing organ prolapse. Organ prolapse is a disorder which occurs when pelvic organs descend into the vaginal or rectal space as a result of weakening of the pelvic floor muscles.

2. Role in Bladder and Bowel Control:

The maintenance of both fecal and urine continence depends heavily on the pelvic floor muscles.

These muscles stay relaxed during regular bladder function to enable efficient voiding. Urine can be released with control when the pelvic floor is engaged, preventing involuntary leaking. In a similar vein, the pelvic floor muscles relax during bowel motions and contract to preserve continence.

3. Importance for Sexual Function and Satisfaction:

Sexual health and pelvic floor health are intimately related. The muscles of the pelvic floor are involved in orgasm and sexual arousal. Enhanced sensation and pleasure during sexual activity are partially attributed to the strength and coordination of the pelvic floor muscles.

While women gain from enhanced vaginal tone, men are linked to healthy pelvic floor function through ejaculatory control and erectile performance.

4. Effect on Core Stability and Posture:

To offer core stability, the deep abdominal and back muscles work in tandem with the pelvic floor muscles. Having a healthy pelvic floor helps one to keep their back straight, support their spine, and avoid problems like lower back discomfort.

To prevent pelvic floor strain, the pelvic floor must be properly engaged during tasks involving lifting and force application.

5. Support During Pregnancy and Childbirth:

The pelvic floor adjusts to the growing weight of the uterus during pregnancy, providing vital support to avoid problems like incontinence.

The pelvic floor's capacity to expand and relax during childbirth is essential for a more seamless delivery experience.

After childbirth, the pelvic floor is important for healing, and specific exercises are frequently advised to rebuild strength.

6. Stability of the Pelvic Girdle:

The stability of the hips and sacrum as well as the entire pelvic girdle depends on the pelvic floor.

This stability helps with overall mobility and balance and is necessary for a variety of actions, such as running, walking, and standing.

7. Regulation of Pressure within the Abdominal Cavity:

Coordinating with the abdominal muscles, the pelvic floor helps regulate intra-abdominal pressure.

For tasks like lifting large things, where a balanced interplay between the pelvic floor and core muscles reduces strain, proper management of pressure is essential.

8. Role in Respiratory Function:

The diaphragm's ability to control breathing patterns is greatly influenced by the pelvic floor.

Coordination of pelvic floor movement with efficient diaphragmatic breathing promotes lung capacity and good respiratory function.

Common Issues Related to Pelvic Floor Dysfunction

1. PELVIC PAIN DISORDERS

Pelvic pain problems are the result of a complicated interaction of psychological, emotional, and physiological elements. Readers will learn more about the unique difficulties caused by pelvic floor tension myalgia, prostatitis, and dyspareunia in this section. Understanding the relationship between these disorders and the pelvic floor will enable readers to examine the function of specific Kegel exercises in the context of an all-encompassing treatment plan.

A. Dyspareunia

Definition: Pain experienced during or after sexual intercourse.

Causes include infections, psychological issues, muscular spasms, and dry vagina.

Pelvic Floor Connection: Pain may be exacerbated by tense pelvic floor muscles.

The function of Kegel exercises: By releasing tension in the muscles, these exercises can help reduce pain.

B. Prostatitis:

Definition: Prostate gland inflammation, which frequently results in pelvic pain.

Causes: Inflammation, tense muscles, and bacterial infection.

Pelvic Floor Connection: Symptoms may worsen if there is tension in the pelvic floor muscles.

The function of Kegel exercises: Kegel exercises play a specific role in strengthening and relaxing the pelvic floor muscles, which may help with symptoms.

C. Tension Myalgia of the Pelvic Floor:

Definition: Chronic pelvic pain related to muscle strain in the pelvic floor.

Causes: Posture problems, trauma, and ongoing stress.

Pelvic Floor Connection: Pain resulting from chronic strain in the muscles of the pelvic floor.

The function of Kegel exercises: Kegel exercises have a key role in releasing tension and regaining equilibrium through gradual, controlled movements.

2. INCONTINENCE

This refers to lack of voluntary control over urination.

Types of Incontinence:

a. Stress Incontinence:

Definition: Unintentional bladder leakage that occurs when performing actions that put strain on the bladder, such as exercising, sneezing, or coughing.

Prevalence: Common in women, especially after childbirth, and also observed in men with compromised pelvic floor muscles.

b. Urge Incontinence:

Definition: An abrupt, strong urge to urinate that frequently results in unintentional urine leakage.

Causes include urinary tract infections, neurological disorders, and overactive bladder muscles.

Impact: May seriously impair quality of life and daily activities.

c. Overflow Incontinence:

Definition: Inability to completely empty the bladder, leading to persistent dribbling or leaking.

Causes: Weak bladder muscles, neurological disorders, or urethral obstruction.

Identifying Symptoms: Constant dribbling, a sense of incomplete evacuation, and recurrent UTIs

Prevalence and Variations by Gender:

- Stress incontinence in women is frequently brought on by pregnancy, childbirth, and hormonal changes.

- Men may experience problems with incontinence following prostate surgery or as they age.

Relation to Weak Muscles of the Pelvic Floor:

- Incontinence is frequently caused by weak pelvic floor muscles.

- Pelvic floor strengthening exercises: Kegel exercises serve as a successful, non-invasive way to strengthen the muscles in the pelvic floor.

3. PELVIC ORGANS PROLAPSE

Definition: Pelvic organ prolapse occurs when pelvic organs, such as the uterus, bladder, or rectum, drop into the vaginal region due to weaker pelvic floor muscles and ligaments.

Causes:

- Childbirth: Trauma during childbirth, especially multiple or painful deliveries.

- Hormonal Shifts and Age: Hormonal changes associated with menopause might damage pelvic tissues.

- Constant constipation or frequent hard lifting are examples of chronic straining.

- Disorders of the Connective Tissues: Affected tissue conditions may be a factor.

- Obesity: Carrying too much weight can put strain on the pelvic muscles and tissues.

Factors related to lifestyle:

- Persistent straining or hefty lifting.

- Persistent coughing.

- Being overweight.

- Genetic factors: Prolapse of the pelvic organs in the family history.

Strengthening Supportive Muscles:

Kegel exercises specifically target and strengthen the pelvic floor muscles that provide support to the pelvic organs.

4. POOR SEXUAL PERFORMANCE

Ineffective sexual performance can be a difficult and delicate problem that has an emotional and physical impact on people and their partners. A comprehensive strategy is needed to address issues around sexual performance, taking into account all of the possible contributing factors.

Factors responsible for poor sexual performance

Physical Factors:

- Lack of Adequate Exercise: Sexual health and physical exercise are intimately related.

Cardiovascular function can be impacted by inactivity, which can alter blood flow to the sexual organs.

- Weak pelvic floor muscles: Weak pelvic floor muscles can also lead to poor sexual performance.

- Medical illnesses: Sexual performance can be affected by a number of medical illnesses, including diabetes, cardiovascular problems, hormonal imbalances, and neurological abnormalities.

- Adverse effects of medication: Arousal, libido, and the capacity to sustain an erection can all be negatively impacted by the side effects of certain drugs.

Psychological factors:

- Stress and Anxiety: Excessive amounts of stress and anxiety, whether brought on by relationships, the workplace, or personal issues, might affect one's ability to perform sexually.

- Performance anxiety can result in subpar performance because of worries about one's capacity to perform sexually or fear of not living up to expectations.

Way of Life and Routines:

Unwise Lifestyle Decisions: Sedentary lifestyles, heavy alcohol use, and smoking are among unhealthy habits that can lead to problems with sexual performance.

CHAPTER TWO

BENEFITS OF KEGEL EXERCISE

Kegel exercises have numerous advantages that improve many facets of health and wellbeing. They include:

1. **Improved Bladder Control:**

- Decrease in Incontinence Incidents: Kegel exercises target and strengthen the pelvic floor muscles, which regulate the flow of urine.

- Urgency and Frequency Reduction: Regular Kegel exercises help improve control over the urge to urinate by lowering the frequency and intensity of unexpected urges. Those with overactive bladder problems will especially benefit from this change.

2. **Enhanced Sexual Performance:**

- Enhanced Sensitivity and Pleasure: During sexual activities, strengthening the pelvic floor can improve blood flow to the vaginal area, which can lead to heightened sensations and heightened sensitivity.

- Improved Blood Flow to the Genital Area: Kegel exercises help to maintain good circulation, which enhances the blood flow to the genital area. Both men and women benefit particularly from this, since it may help with erectile dysfunction and improve general sexual function.

- Treating Erectile Dysfunction and Premature Ejaculation: By encouraging improved control over the pelvic floor muscles, a regimen that includes Kegel exercises for men may help address problems associated with erectile dysfunction and premature ejaculation.

3. **Pelvic organ prolapse prevention and management:**

Building up Supportive Muscles: Pelvic organ prolapse is the result of the pelvic floor becoming weaker, which permits the uterus, bladder, or rectum to drop. By strengthening the supporting muscles, Kegel exercises function prophylactically, possibly avoiding or lessening prolapse.

4. Relieving Pelvic Pain:

Relaxation and Release of Tension: Pelvic pain syndromes, including dyspareunia and tension myalgia, commonly include muscular tension. Kegel exercises, when performed properly, can aid to the relaxation and release of tension in the pelvic floor muscles.

HOW TO DO KEGEL EXERCISES

Locating the pelvic floor muscles

You can identify the pelvic floor muscles by trying to halt the flow of urine. The pelvic floor muscles are the ones you employ for this movement. Get used to how they feel when they contract and relax.

This approach should only be used for educational purposes, though. Regularly starting and stopping your urination or performing Kegel exercises when your bladder is full are not recommended practices. An incomplete bladder emptying can increase your risk of UTIs, or urinary tract infections.

When sitting on the toilet, you can also feel for the pelvic floor muscle by imagining that you are trying to stop gas from passing through. This motion uses muscles that are also a part of the pelvic floor.

For the female, you can also locate your pelvic muscle by placing a clean finger inside your vagina and tightening your vaginal muscles around your finger, while for men, another way to find them is to insert a finger into the rectum and try to squeeze it — without tightening the muscles of the abdomen, buttocks, or thighs.

Steps in doing Kegel exercises

Once you are familiar with the pelvic floor muscles, perform kegel exercises via the following steps:

- Ensure that your bladder is empty before sitting or lying down.

- Sit comfortably, with your back straight or slightly bent inwards

- Squeeze the pelvic floor muscles (the muscle around your anal opening; the muscle around your vaginal opening, and the muscle around the urethral opening) simultaneously and pull them inwardly and wait three to five seconds.

- Release the muscles

- Rest for 6 – 10 seconds between each exercise

- Take deep breaths and keep your body relaxed while performing these exercises.

- Verify that you are not contracting the muscles in your chest, thighs, buttocks, or stomach.

- Repeat the exercise 2 – 3 times per day

- Perform the exercise on most days of the week

Some Basic Points to Note:

How many and for how long?

It's normal to find that your first few attempts only allow you to hold a kegel for three to six seconds, and that performing three to six repetitions wears out your muscles. Usually, you are doing the exercise correctly when this occurs. Recheck your technique if you notice that you can hold it for a longer period of time straight immediately. For patients with incontinence or pelvic floor weakness, it is crucial to focus on doing the method correctly. Your muscles may be weak when you first start training and get stronger over time.

Including Kegels in your daily routine:

Once you've gotten comfortable with these workouts, you should perform them as follows:

- A set of eight to ten strong, continuous squeezes, performed eight to ten at a time, thirty times a day

As they become easier, you'll discover that you can perform them both sitting and standing—for instance, while operating a vehicle, using a computer, or standing in line.

Note that it can take some time before you notice any change in your ability to regulate your bladder or bowels. Sometimes, it could take many months.

Note:

When performing the exercises, keep in mind to:

• Keep breathing while doing the exercises

• Eat fruit and vegetables; • Drink six to eight glasses of water a day; • Relax your thighs; • Avoid straining when using the restroom; • Maintain a weight that is appropriate for your age and height.

Try not to overdo the exercises:

Avoid performing more than 100 Kegel exercises in a single day as this may cause muscle fatigue and increased leakage. Start out slowly and raise the quantity of exercise over time.

Breathe during the exercises, don't forget. Your pelvic muscles may experience increased pressure if you hold your breath.

Consistent practice helps build muscle memory and gradually strengthens the pelvic floor.

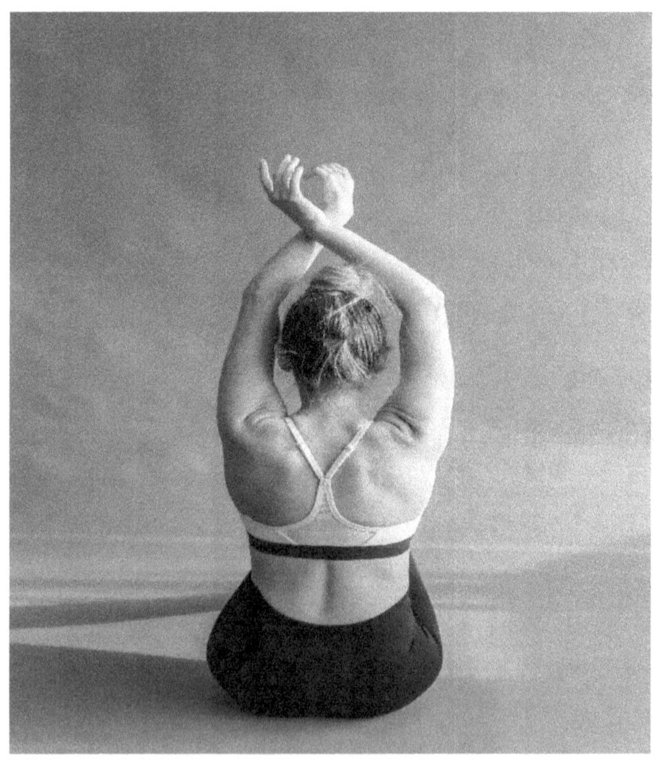

CHAPTER THREE

SPECIAL CONCERNS FOR WOMEN

Kegel Exercises During Pregnancy

Performing Kegel exercises when pregnant has enormous advantages. They include:

a. **Better Pelvic Floor Support:** The body changes significantly throughout pregnancy to make room for the developing fetus. There is more pressure on the pelvic floor. Kegel exercises help to strengthen these muscles, which in turn helps to maintain general pelvic stability and improves support for the developing uterus. As the pregnancy goes on, this support becomes increasingly important in preventing problems like pelvic organ prolapse and incontinence.

b. Lower Risk of Incontinence: Some women may experience urine incontinence as a result of hormonal changes and the physical strain of pregnancy. Kegel exercises promote greater strength and control by focusing on the muscles involved in bladder control. Because of this, women who consistently perform Kegel exercises during pregnancy may have a lower chance of developing urine incontinence during and after giving birth.

c. Labor and Delivery Preparation: Due to their potential to ease labor and delivery, Kegel exercises are frequently advised as part of prenatal preparation. Enhancing pelvic floor muscular strength can help better regulate and focus pushing forces during childbirth. Furthermore, preserving the pelvic floor's strength and flexibility may facilitate a more seamless postpartum recuperation.

These advantages highlight how crucial it is to incorporate Kegel exercises into the pregnant routine for the pelvic floor's long-term health as well as for immediate comfort. Maintaining a regular routine during pregnancy can help provide the groundwork for a successful postpartum recovery and make giving birth more enjoyable.

When to Begin Kegel Exercises While Expectant:

A. The First Trimester: Laying the Groundwork

Women can start laying the groundwork for a basic grasp of Kegel exercises during their first trimester.

To familiarize the pelvic floor muscles with the exercise, there should be a focus on mild contractions and releases.

Early involvement promotes awareness of the pelvic floor's function throughout pregnancy and aids in the establishment of a mind-body link.

B. Modifying Intensity in the Second and Third Trimesters:

The intensity of Kegel exercises can be modified as the pregnancy goes on.

To progressively improve pelvic floor strength, longer contractions and more deliberate releases should be used.

To enhance general wellbeing, concentrate on implementing Kegel exercises into a thorough pregnancy exercise program.

Kegel exercises can be started in the first trimester, which permits a methodical and gradual approach to pelvic floor health. The workouts change as the pregnancy goes on to meet the body's evolving needs. The ideal preparation for the physical demands of delivery and postpartum recovery is facilitated by the growing intensity and integration of these activities with other prenatal activities. Crucially, before beginning any fitness program, expectant mothers should always speak with their healthcare providers to be sure it is appropriate for their unique health concerns and the stage of their pregnancy.

Safe Practices for Kegels During Pregnancy:

A. Modified Positions for Comfort:

The body's changing anatomy during pregnancy might affect how accessible and comfortable workouts, including Kegel exercises, are. This section emphasizes how important it is to use positions that have been adapted to meet the special requirements of expectant mothers in order to maximize comfort and efficacy.

Changing with Your Body: Expectant mothers should be aware of their bodies, seeing how their weight changes and their posture alters during pregnancy.

Considering Flexibility: It is crucial to modify positions to account for any restrictions or pain brought on by variations in range of motion or flexibility.

Positions for Sitting and Side-Lying: It is advised to practice Kegel exercises while seated in order to reduce tension on the lower back and relieve pressure on the abdomen.

Kegel exercises that require side lying are recommended in order to target the pelvic floor muscles and offer extra support and comfort, especially in the later stages of pregnancy.

Lumbar Support: To help maintain optimal spinal alignment and lessen pressure on the lower back, promote the usage of pillows for lumbar support when seated.

Under Hip Support: To enhance comfort and help align the pelvis and relieve pressure during side-lying Kegel exercises, it is recommended to place a pillow under the hip.

Including Mild Stretches: To enhance flexibility and relieve any tension in the surrounding muscles, it is recommended to perform mild stretching exercises both prior to and following Kegel exercises.

Warm-up Methods: Provide pelvic-focused warm-up methods to facilitate a smooth and comfortable transition into the exercises.

Promoting Self-Monitoring: Any discomfort or strain should be quickly attended to, and different positions should be investigated.

Individualized Approach: Recognize that the comfort level of different positions varies across persons; consequently, supporting an individualized approach to meet personal preferences and needs.

Frequent Body Check-ins: Expectant mothers should regularly assess their level of comfort during physical activity by performing body check-ins. Changes or breaks can be made as needed if pain or strain develops.

B. Steer clear of strain and overexertion:

Preventing strain and overexertion is a crucial component of performing Kegel exercises properly when pregnant. Due to the substantial physiological changes that occur during pregnancy, it is imperative that pelvic floor exercises be performed mindfully and methodically. In-depth instructions on identifying and avoiding strain during Kegel exercises for various stages of pregnancy are provided in this section.

Recognizing Physical Limits: The body experiences many changes throughout pregnancy, such as hormone changes, weight growth, and postural adjustments. The pelvic floor muscles may be affected by these alterations. The physical boundaries that these changes impose must be recognized and respected. The basis for safe Kegel exercises is the knowledge that pregnant women should have that their bodies are changing to accommodate the growing baby.

Keeping an Eye Out for Overexertion: When doing Kegel exercises while pregnant, overexertion can result in weariness, pain, or even injury. It is recommended that women pay close attention to cues from their body, such as pressure in the pelvic area, aches in the muscles, or overall exhaustion. To avoid putting yourself under unnecessary strain, it's critical to adjust or stop the workouts if any of these symptoms appear.

Changing the Intensity of the Exercise: Adapting the Kegel exercises to your own level of discomfort is essential. Being pregnant is a dynamic process, so something that is easy in one trimester could be difficult in another. To reduce tension, modifications could include shortening the workout sessions, changing the amount of repetitions, or using kinder alternatives.

C.   Nutrition and Hydration:

When it comes to safe Kegel exercise routines during pregnancy, maintaining general health and, by extension, pelvic floor function, requires careful consideration of nutrition and hydration. The importance of eating a balanced diet and staying properly hydrated is discussed in this subsection in order to maximize the benefits of Kegel exercises.

Highlighting Appropriate Hydration:

Because of things like increased blood volume and amniotic fluid, pregnancy raises the body's fluid requirements. Maintaining adequate hydration is essential for general health, which includes pelvic floor muscle function.

Improving the Performance of Muscles: Muscles that are well-hydrated are more flexible and perform at their best. The flexibility and reactivity of the pelvic floor muscles are supported by adequate water intake, which enhances the efficacy of Kegel exercises.

Keeping Dehydration-Related Pain at Bay: Constipation and urinary tract problems are among the discomforts that can result from dehydration. Pregnant women can lessen their chances of experiencing these discomforts by drinking enough water, which will improve the environment for pelvic exercises.

A Well-Balanced Diet for Pregnancy: During pregnancy, the strength and resiliency of muscles, particularly the pelvic floor, are greatly impacted by the quality of nourishment received.

Fiber and Healthy Digestive System: During pregnancy, constipation is a major problem that can worsen pelvic floor discomfort. A high-fiber diet encourages regular bowel movements, which eases pelvic floor pressure and enhances the benefits of Kegel exercises.

Steer Clear of Too Much Sugar and Caffeine: Consuming too much sugar and caffeine can cause dehydration and negatively affect pelvic health. For the sake of your general health, encourage moderation when ingesting these substances.

Custom Kegel Exercises for Postpartum Recuperation:

The pelvic floor alters significantly after childbirth. It is essential to comprehend these modifications in order to properly customize Kegel exercises. Postpartum pelvic health is shaped by various factors, including muscular laxity, possible tearing, and the effect of delivery modalities (by vaginal birth or C-section).

Reintroducing Kegel Exercises Gradually:

The postpartum body goes through an amazing healing process, therefore it's important to go cautiously while reintroducing Kegel exercises. This stage offers a planned method for progressively reinstating Kegel exercises while also acknowledging the particular difficulties faced by women during postpartum recovery.

Early Postpartum Phase:

The emphasis during the first several days after giving birth is on rest and recuperation. Kegel exercises are gradually introduced, emphasizing minimal muscular activation and regulated breathing. The purpose of this first stage is to connect with the pelvic floor muscles without overstressing the body.

Evaluation of the Pelvic Floor:

Women are advised to self-evaluate their pelvic floor before beginning a regular Kegel program. This include locating any sore spots, weak points, or knots. Kegel exercise modifications are based on an understanding of the pelvic floor's current condition and target individual needs.

Considering Comfort Levels:

Kegel exercise reintroduction is based on each person's comfort level. It is advised that women begin with brief, mild contractions and progressively increase the length and force when they feel ready. Keeping an eye out for any indications of pain guarantees a secure and efficient advancement.

Keeping an Eye Out for Indices of Stress or Unease:

Women are advised to keep an eye out for any indications of strain or discomfort during the gradual reintroduction. It's critical to distinguish between any signs of overexertion and the typical feelings brought on by muscle activity. Changes are implemented in response to individual input.

Frequent Check-ins and Assessment of Progress:

It is recommended to regularly check in to assess progress. It is advised that women think back on their experiences and record any shifts in their strength, comfort, or general well-being. These check-ins help with the continuous modification of the Kegel regimen to meet changing postpartum requirements.

Customizing Kegels for Scar Tissue Healing:

Understanding the Impact of Scar Tissue: After childbirth, particularly in cases of perineal tearing or C-sections, the formation of scar tissue is common. This scar tissue can affect the flexibility and mobility of the pelvic floor muscles. Understanding the impact of scar tissue is crucial in tailoring Kegel exercises for effective healing.

1. **Identifying Scar Tissue:**

- Begin by identifying the location and extent of the scar tissue. Women can gently explore the area, both visually and through touch, to locate any areas of tenderness or stiffness. Awareness of scar tissue helps in customizing Kegel exercises to address specific concerns.

2. **Gentle Massage Techniques:**

- Incorporate gentle massage techniques to promote blood flow and flexibility around the scar tissue. Before initiating Kegel exercises, women can use their fingers or a specialized massaging tool to apply gentle pressure to the scar area. This aids in breaking down adhesions and reducing discomfort.

3. **Targeted Kegel Contractions:**

- Once the scar tissue is identified and massaged, integrate targeted Kegel contractions that focus on the affected area. Customizing Kegels involves engaging the pelvic floor muscles while paying specific attention to the scar tissue. These targeted contractions help in strengthening and promoting healing in the scarred region.

4.   **Gradual Progression:**

- Customization also involves a gradual progression of intensity. Start with light contractions, gradually increasing the engagement of the pelvic floor muscles over time. This step-by-step approach allows the scar tissue to adapt and heal without causing unnecessary strain.

5.   **Monitoring Discomfort Levels:**

- Regularly monitor discomfort levels during and after customized Kegel exercises. It's normal to experience mild discomfort initially, but persistent pain or increased discomfort may indicate the need for adjustments. Listening to one's body and adjusting the routine accordingly is key to a safe and effective recovery.

CHAPTER FOUR

SPECIAL CONCERNS FOR MEN

Benefits of Kegel Exercise for Men

Kegel exercises, which are frequently linked to women's health, are also very important for men's sexual health. The pelvic floor muscles, which support many body functions, including those connected to sexual performance, are the focus of these workouts. The advantages of Kegel exercises for men's sexual health are examined in detail below:

A. Effect of Kegel Exercise on the Prostate Gland

Understanding the complex interaction between the pelvic floor muscles and the prostate gland is essential to using Kegel exercises to address prostate health. The prostate, a little gland the size of a walnut that is located around the urethra and behind the bladder, is essential to the health of male reproduction. Kegel exercises can be included into a program to provide a number of advantages for keeping the prostate healthy:

Improved Circulation of Blood:

Kegel exercises work the pelvic floor muscles by contracting and relaxing them, which increases blood flow to the pelvic area. By guaranteeing that the prostate gland receives a constant supply of oxygen and nutrients, improved blood flow can support improved prostate health.

Building Up the Pelvic Floor Muscles:

The prostate and other pelvic organs are supported by the muscles of the pelvic floor. Kegel exercises that strengthen these muscles support the prostate and help keep the pelvic region structurally intact, preventing problems like enlargement or drooping.

Diminished Prostate Symptoms:

Urinary urgency, frequency, or difficulty are signs of some prostate disorders, such as prostatitis or benign prostatic hyperplasia (BPH). Frequent Kegel exercises can help reduce these symptoms by improving pelvic floor muscle control and coordination, which improves urine function.

Preventing Enlargement of the Prostate:

Benign prostatic hyperplasia (BPH) is a disorder where men's prostate gland enlarges with age. Although Kegel exercises are unlikely to prevent BPH outright, they can help keep the prostate healthy by strengthening the surrounding pelvic muscles and possibly reducing symptoms related to enlargement of the prostate.

Support for the Healing of the Prostate:

Men who have prostate-related surgery, such as a prostatectomy, may develop weaker muscles in their pelvis. Kegel exercises are a useful part of the post-surgery rehabilitation regimen because they help strengthen and function the pelvic floor, which promotes overall prostate health.

Encouragement of Prostate Massage:

Flexibility and strength in the pelvic floor muscles are beneficial for prostate massage, a therapeutic method.

Kegel exercises can help make prostate massage more successful by guaranteeing that the pelvic floor is receptive and making the massage procedure easier.

Enhanced Bladder Management:

Urinary incontinence can occasionally be caused by prostate problems. Kegel exercises that strengthen the pelvic floor help improve bladder control, lowering the risk of leaks and improving general urinary health.

Beneficial Effect on Sexual Performance:

Prostate health is essential for preserving sexual function. Kegel exercises can have a good impact on sexual health by strengthening the pelvic floor muscles and increasing blood circulation. This may lead to improvements in ejaculatory control and erectile function.

B. Enhanced Male erection:

Kegel exercises help to increase the pelvic region's blood flow. Since proper blood flow is necessary to achieve and sustain erections, this improved circulation is especially advantageous for erectile function.

Strengthened Pelvic Floor: By giving stability to the surrounding structures, a strong pelvic floor aids in the erectile process. Kegel exercises, which strengthen these muscles, have a beneficial effect on erectile function.

C. Enhanced Control of Ejaculation:

Muscular Endurance: Kegel exercises aim to improve the pelvic floor muscles' endurance. Greater control over the time of ejaculation is made possible by this superior regulation of the ejaculatory reflex, which is a result of the higher muscle control.

Delaying Ejaculation: The capacity to postpone ejaculation has been linked to regular Kegel exercise practice. For men who ejaculate early, building strength in their pelvic floor may help them become more sexually energetic.

D. Enhanced Sensation:

During sexual action, strengthening the pelvic floor may result in heightened sensations. Increased pleasure and satisfaction during a sexual encounter may be a result of improved muscle tone and control.

Improved Orgasmic Response: Kegel exercises may have a beneficial effect on orgasm quality. Men who have stronger pelvic floor muscles may have more satisfying and powerful orgasms.

Confidence in Sexual Performance: Having actively worked to enhance one's sexual health through Kegel exercises might help one feel more confident when having sex.

Increased Body Awareness: One of the benefits of Kegel exercises is an increased awareness of the pelvic floor muscles. Having more awareness might help you be more responsive and in control when engaging in sexual activity.

CHAPTER FIVE
BEYOND KEGELS: COMPLEMENTARY TECHNIQUES

There is a world of supplementary exercises outside Kegels that, when incorporated into your regimen, can enhance the advantages of pelvic floor exercises. These all-encompassing methods, which focus on different facets of general health and wellbeing, complement Kegels. Let's investigate these supplementary methods:

Pelvic Floor Health with Yoga:

Particular Poses: Include poses from yoga that work the pelvic floor, like bound angle pose (Bound Angle Pose), chair pose (Utkatasana), and yoga's Malasana (Yogic Squat).

Breathing Techniques: In yoga, mindful breathing techniques, particularly diaphragmatic breathing, can increase pelvic floor awareness and encourage relaxation.

Core and Pilates Exercises: By giving the muscles surrounding the pelvic floor more support, Pilates exercises, which emphasize core strength, can be used in conjunction with Kegel exercises.

Pilates places a strong emphasis on coordination and control, which benefits both men and women's pelvic floor health by enhancing general body awareness.

Mind-Body Connection: Activities that strengthen the mind-body connection, such as mindfulness and meditation, encourage relaxation and lower stress levels, which may be linked to pelvic floor tightness.

Stress management: Prolonged stress can impair the function of the pelvic floor. Stress can be lessened by practices like mindfulness, meditation, and deep breathing.

Acupuncture: Acupuncture is a part of Traditional Chinese Medicine, which may help balance and enhance energy flow, which may be beneficial to the health of the pelvic floor.

Ergonomics: To avoid putting undue strain on the pelvic floor, practice proper posture, especially when sitting.

Pelvic Alignment: Pelvic misalignment can be treated with techniques such as chiropractic adjustments or osteopathic consultations, which will improve the health of the pelvic floor.

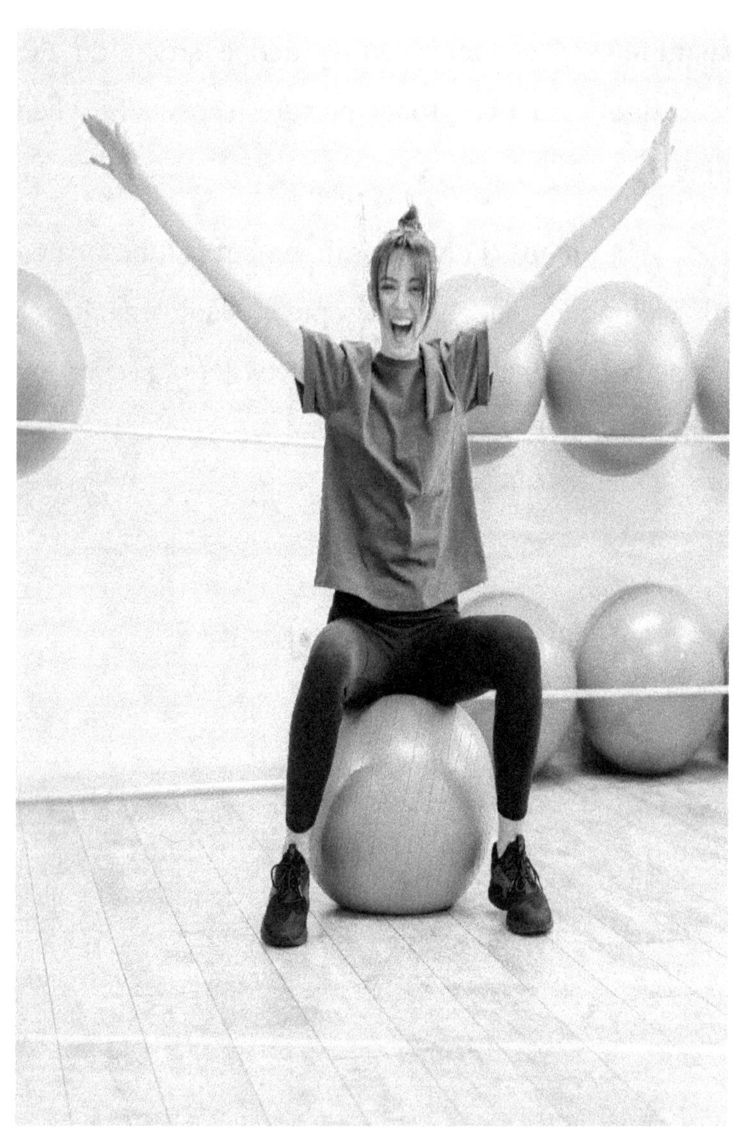

CHAPTER SIX

TRACKING PROGRESS AND ADJUSTING THE ROUTINE

Tracking progress is a pivotal aspect of any exercise regimen, and Kegel exercises are no exception. Monitoring changes in strength, endurance, and any associated symptoms can provide valuable insights into the effectiveness of the routine. Here's an extensive exploration of how to track progress and make necessary adjustments:

A. **Developing a Monitoring System**

1. **Journaling and Logging:**

- Maintain a Kegel exercise journal. This can include details such as the type and duration of exercises, any discomfort or pain experienced, and specific times when exercises were performed.

- Logging daily routines allows for a comprehensive overview of progress over time.

2. **Symptom Tracking:**

- Note any changes in symptoms related to pelvic floor health, such as improvements in bladder control, reduction in pelvic pain, or enhanced sexual satisfaction.

- Record instances of leakage or discomfort to identify patterns and trends.

3. **Strength Assessment:**

- Periodically reassess pelvic floor strength using self-assessment tools or seeking guidance from a healthcare professional.

- Evaluate the ease with which you can control and contract your pelvic floor muscles.

B. **Recognizing Positive Changes**

1. **Improved Control:**

- Acknowledge any enhancements in the ability to contract and relax pelvic floor muscles. Improved control is a positive sign of strengthening.

- Celebrate achievements in achieving longer contraction durations or more repetitions over time.

2. **Reduced Symptoms:**

- Highlight reductions in symptoms associated with pelvic floor dysfunction, such as decreased frequency of urinary incontinence or alleviation of pelvic pain.

- Pay attention to improvements in sexual function, including enhanced arousal or ejaculatory control.

3. **Enhanced Daily Functioning:**

- Recognize how strengthened pelvic floor muscles positively impact daily activities, from more effortless movement to increased comfort during prolonged periods of sitting.

C. Modifying Exercises Based on Progress

1. Increasing Intensity:

- Gradually progress to more advanced exercises as strength improves. This may involve incorporating resistance, increasing the duration of contractions, or adding variations to challenge the muscles further.

- Make sure to maintain proper form and technique during more challenging exercises.

2. **Adjusting Frequency:**

- Evaluate the current exercise frequency and make adjustments based on progress. As strength increases, you may reduce the frequency of basic exercises while incorporating more advanced routines.

3. **Consistent Self-Assessment:**

- Be consistent in self-assessing your progress. Regularly revisit journal entries, reassess strength, and adjust routines accordingly.

- Ongoing self-awareness is key to maintaining and continually improving pelvic floor health.

CONCLUSION

These pages aren't the only places where Kegels' magic exists. It's inside you, just waiting to be let go. What comes next, then? Will you be the pelvic floor's champion, spending just a few minutes a day harnessing its power? Will you impart this information to others, turning yourself into a source of empowerment? Decide to stand up, take ownership of your pelvic health, and radiate Kegels' magic. The world is eagerly awaiting your distinct kind of pelvic strength. Are you prepared to let it loose?